Phoebe the Pug asks

"Is my Asthma Changing?"

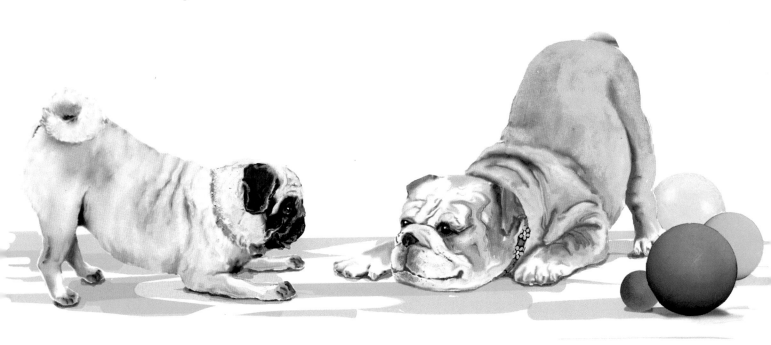

Dr. Donna Jean Matlach

Copyright 2017 – Dr. Donna Jean Matlach

Published by: Dr. Donna Jean Matlach

Email: drdonnajeanmatlach@gmail.com
Tel: 623-252-1230

Cover design & illustrations: Dr. Carrie Wachsmann (professional author & artist)
Editor: Mai-Ly Duong, DMD, MPH, MAEd (healthcare professional & educator)

ISBN #: 978-1974065332
Printed in USA

The opinions of this book are solely those of the author. Medical care is highly individualized and should never be altered without professional medical consultation.

To order additional copies of this book or inquire about our quantity discounts for schools, hospitals, and affiliated organizations, please contact us directly at the information listed above.

ACKNOWLEDGEMENTS

*God has blessed me with people in my life
who have helped me and held me up
when I was not able to do it on my own.
Thank you and God Bless You.*

Charles A. Matlach, DDS, MM – my wonderful husband

Mai-Ly Duong, DMD, MPH, MAEd – my dear friend

Mark S. Forshag, MD, MHA
US Medical Expert – Respiratory, North American Medical Affairs

Karen Drake, D.Min. – President, Primus University of Theology
(previously Phoenix University of Theology)

Kristin R. Risch, MSEd

Nick Risch, MS

Deanna M. Rizzotto

Tonya Winders – CEO & President, Allergy & Asthma Network

Introduction

Dear Readers,

Not all asthma is the same.
Having asthma does not make someone abnormal or different.

Asthma may present itself in many forms and severities. It is important to be aware that asthma can affect anyone, anywhere. It transcends all age, race, gender, and socioeconomic levels.

Thank you for allowing me the opportunity to share this beautiful story with you. The main character in this story, Phoebe the Pug, is a courageous young pup, who faces many physical, emotional, and social challenges due to her asthma.

I hope that this story helps all of us demonstrate compassion and understanding for those who have illnesses that significantly change and influence their lives.

All my best,
Donna Jean Matlach

Dedication

First, to my Lord, Jesus Christ, who has given me life AND a second chance at it. He has made me sensitive to the needs of others and filled me with compassion and love, in word, thought and deed.

Second, to my husband, Charlie, who has given endlessly of his love and himself, taking care of me.

To my incredible friend, Mai-Ly, who has taught me to "breathe" even when I think I can't.

Momma – Thank you for loving me and encouraging me to "Reach for the stars!" and holding my hand every step of the way! YOU ARE MY HERO! I LOVE YOU!

And to my daughters and granddaughters, I love you to the moon and back…. And a bazillion times more than all the fish in the sea, and the sand on the beaches, and the stars in the sky, and to infinity and beyond!!!!

DIIIING! The school bell rings.

Mrs. Shepherd, the teacher, happily says,
"It's time for recess, everyone!"

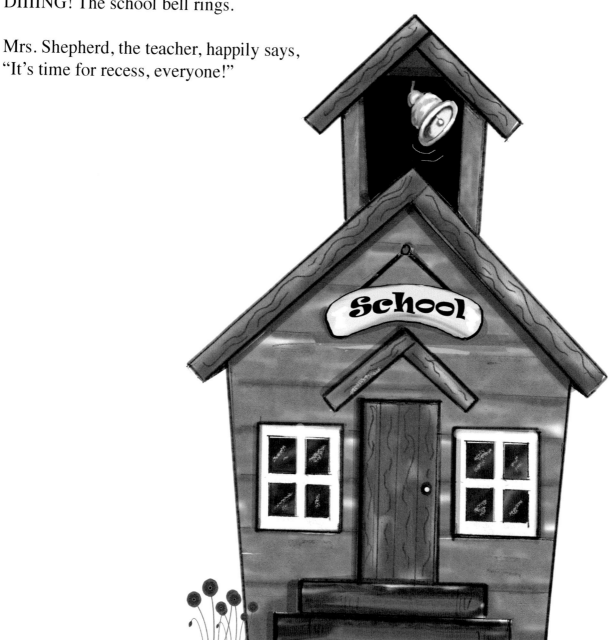

Phoebe the Pug quickly grabs her rescue inhaler from her desk and takes a big puff, as instructed by her doctor before she goes out to play. She is looking forward to playing with the other puppies at recess.

As the other pups run out of the room and onto the playground, she tries her best to keep up with them. When she finally reaches the other pups, she starts to feel her chest tighten and begins to gasp for air.

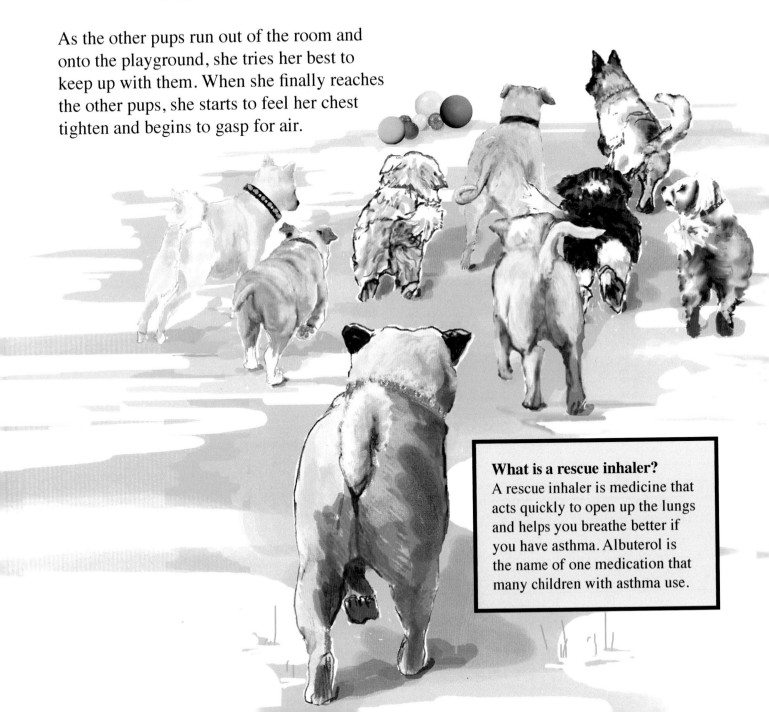

What is a rescue inhaler?
A rescue inhaler is medicine that acts quickly to open up the lungs and helps you breathe better if you have asthma. Albuterol is the name of one medication that many children with asthma use.

After a few moments and a bit of a scare, she finally catches her breath. She reaches the other puppies but is still coughing.

Despite the coughing, Phoebe barks, "Hey guys, can I play fetch with you, too?"

Everyone looks at each other and then stares at her.

Then Bina the Bulldog yells, "No, we don't want to play with you. You're sick! We don't want to get what you have!" The pups run away, leaving Phoebe behind.

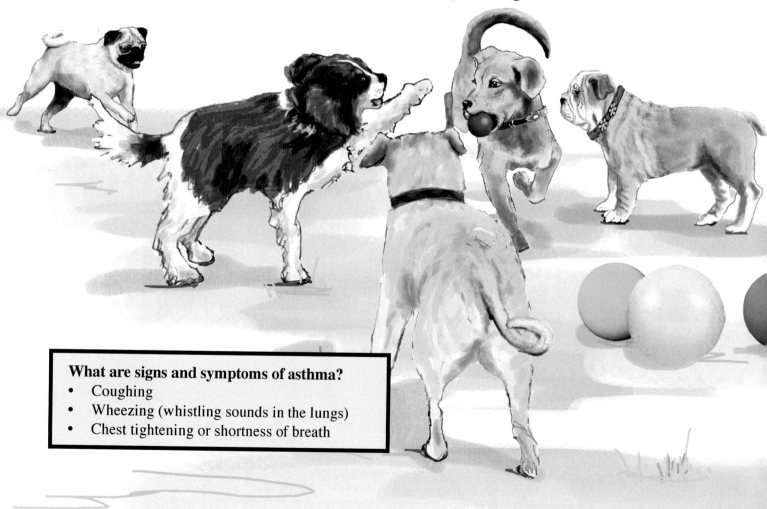

What are signs and symptoms of asthma?
- Coughing
- Wheezing (whistling sounds in the lungs)
- Chest tightening or shortness of breath

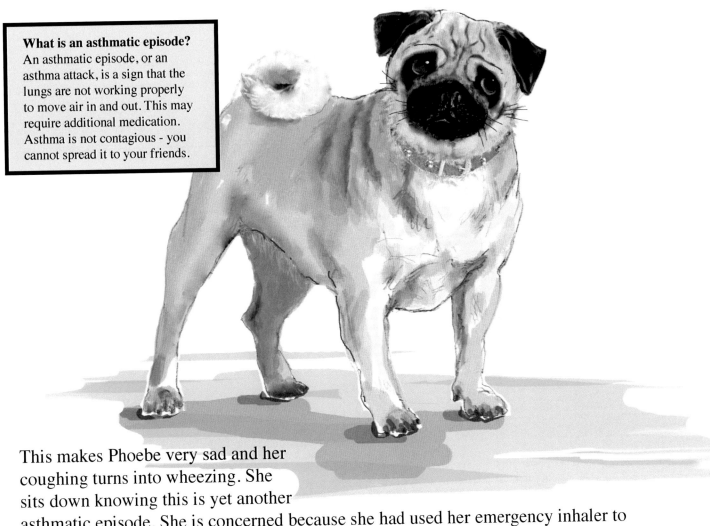

This makes Phoebe very sad and her coughing turns into wheezing. She sits down knowing this is yet another asthmatic episode. She is concerned because she had used her emergency inhaler to help her breathe just a few minutes ago. Phoebe remembers her doctor telling her she should not need her emergency inhaler so often.

A few minutes go by, and her wheezing goes away. Phoebe decides she would like to try to play with the other pups again. She jumps up and runs out to the field. As she gets closer to the pups, she slows down because she cannot catch her breath again. The pups stop playing and stare at her. Then Bina says, "Go away, you're contagious – we could get what you have!"

9

Suddenly, the bell "DINGS" again, and all the pups start running back to class without helping Phoebe.

As Phoebe the Pug slowly approaches the classroom by herself, Mrs. Shepherd, her teacher, notices Phoebe struggling to breathe and says quietly, "Phoebe, why don't you go to the nurse's office to get a breathing treatment?"

Phoebe listens and turns towards the nurse's office.

What can others do when someone has an asthmatic episode?
When someone has an asthmatic episode, they may need medicine like an inhaler or a breathing treatment. It is important not to leave them alone. It is also important to find someone who can help.

Phoebe has been spending a lot of time at the nurse's office lately.

There is always a comfortable place for Phoebe to rest when she visits. This is also where she receives her breathing treatment with the nebulizer. Mr. Dachshund is the nicest nurse in the world.

Mr. Dachsund puts a small mask over Phoebe's nose, and she begins breathing in the mist. The medicine in the mist makes her airways open up so air can get in and help her feel better!

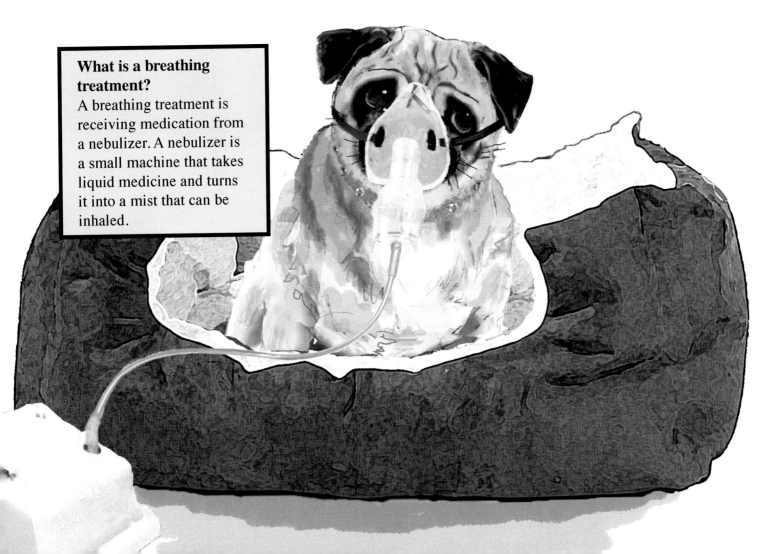

What is a breathing treatment?
A breathing treatment is receiving medication from a nebulizer. A nebulizer is a small machine that takes liquid medicine and turns it into a mist that can be inhaled.

Once she can breathe normally again, Mr. Dachshund says to her, "Phoebe, this is the third day in a row that you have needed to use the nebulizer treatment. I think you should see a breathing specialist called a pulmonologist. His name is Dr. Dalmatian. You should go see him tomorrow to figure out why you are getting asthmatic episodes more often than usual."

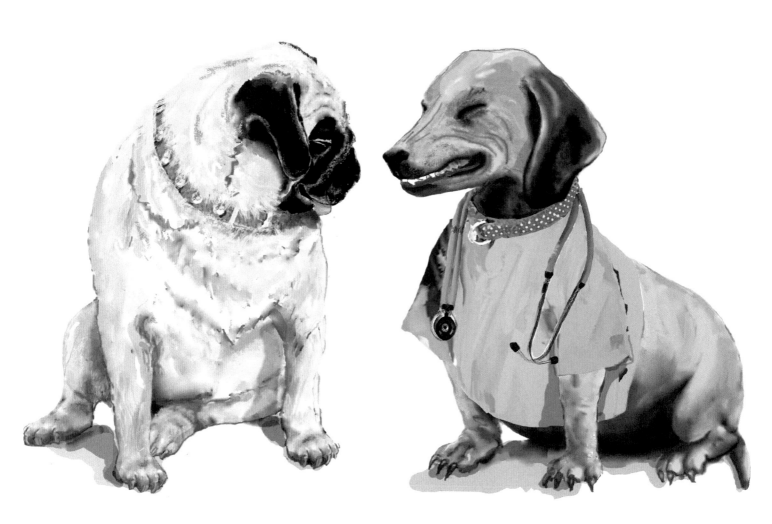

Feeling better, Phoebe marches back to class and sits down.

On her desk, she finds a note that reads, "Go Home. You're contagious! We don't like to play with sick pups."

Phoebe looks up and finds Bina the Bulldog staring right at her with a scowl. Phoebe becomes even more embarrassed and uncomfortable. She sits quietly for the rest of the day and then walks home by herself as soon as school is over.

Is asthma contagious?
No, asthma is not contagious. You cannot catch asthma from others. People with asthma are normal just like everyone else.

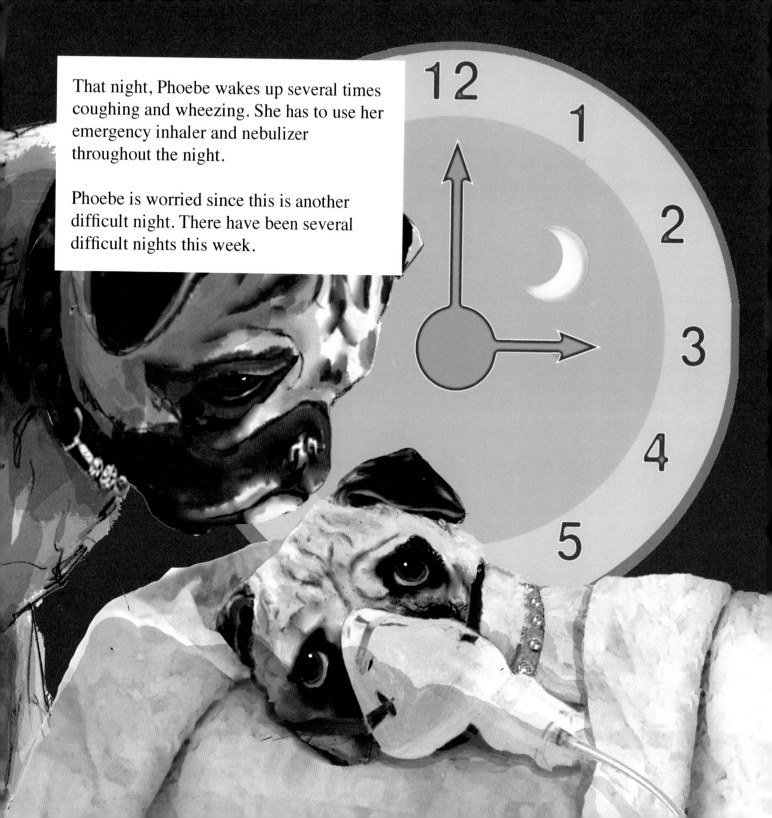

That night, Phoebe wakes up several times coughing and wheezing. She has to use her emergency inhaler and nebulizer throughout the night.

Phoebe is worried since this is another difficult night. There have been several difficult nights this week.

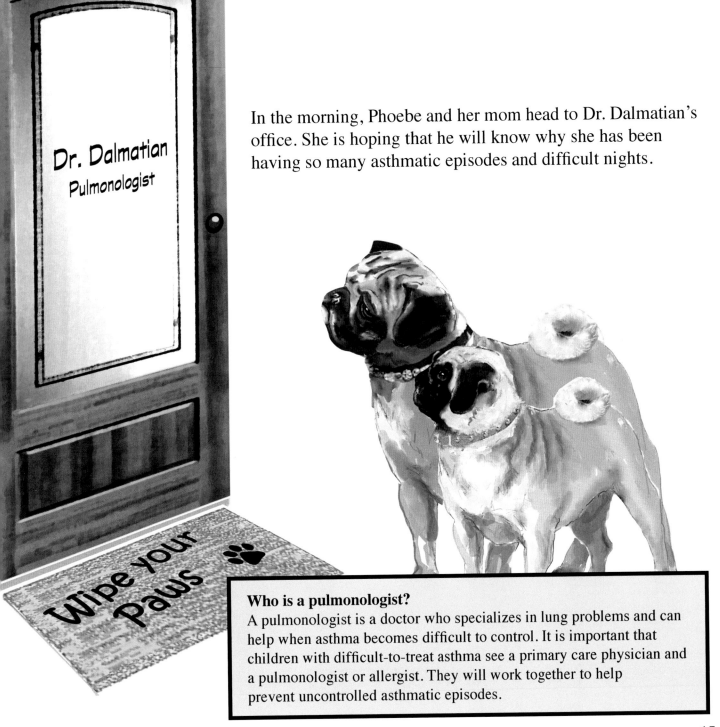

Dr. Dalmatian
Pulmonologist

Wipe your Paws

In the morning, Phoebe and her mom head to Dr. Dalmatian's office. She is hoping that he will know why she has been having so many asthmatic episodes and difficult nights.

Who is a pulmonologist?
A pulmonologist is a doctor who specializes in lung problems and can help when asthma becomes difficult to control. It is important that children with difficult-to-treat asthma see a primary care physician and a pulmonologist or allergist. They will work together to help prevent uncontrolled asthmatic episodes.

15

At school, the pups definitely notice that Phoebe is not in class, and rumors begin to circulate about why Phoebe is not there.

Bina the Bulldog comments, "I'm glad she stayed home so we don't get sick."

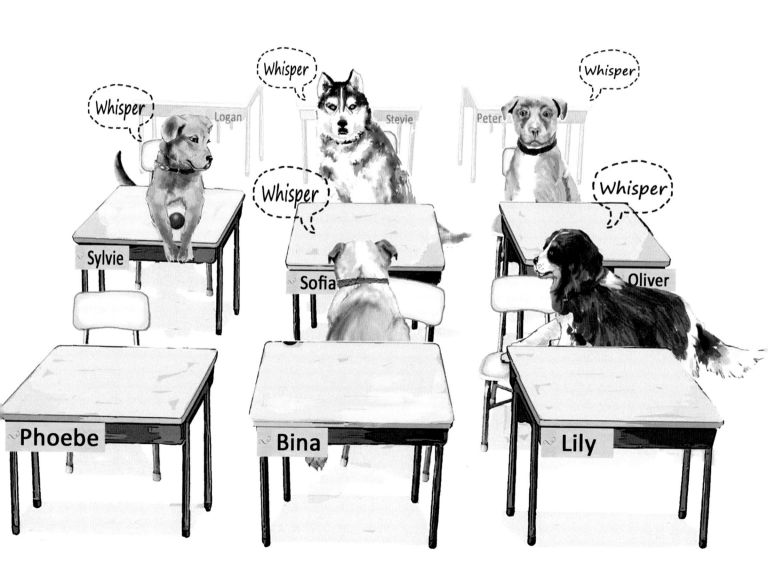

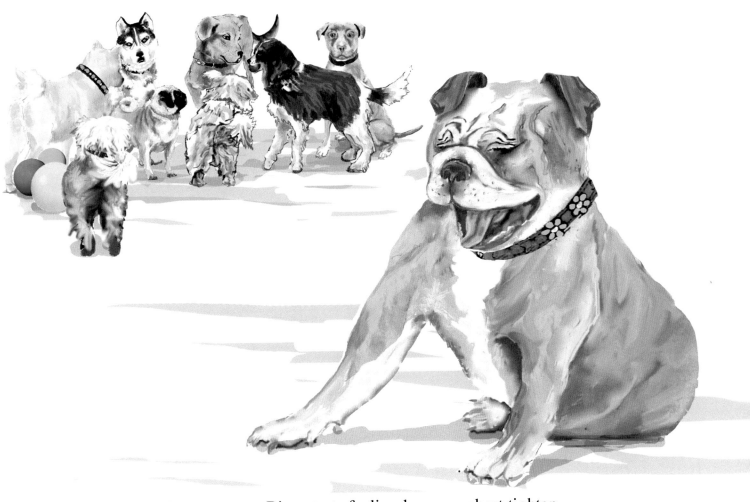

That day at recess, Bina starts feeling her own chest tighten.

As she frolics with the rest of the pups playing fetch, she also begins to have shortness of breath. Then suddenly, *she* starts coughing!

The other pups say, "Oh no! You're sick too! We don't want to play with you anymore!"

Bina's coughing gets worse. This scares her, and she quickly goes to the nurse's office.

Mr. Dachshund listens to Bina's lungs. He says that although her breathing returned to normal, he does hear some wheezing in her lungs.

Mr. Dachshund says that she should see the pulmonologist, Dr. Dalmatian, as soon as possible. He also tells her that she might need a rescue inhaler if she has more trouble breathing.

A few minutes later, her father picks her up from school and takes her to Dr. Dalmatian's office.

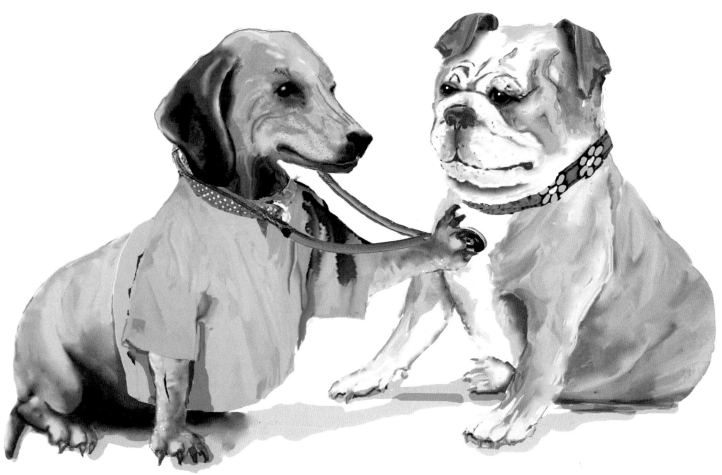

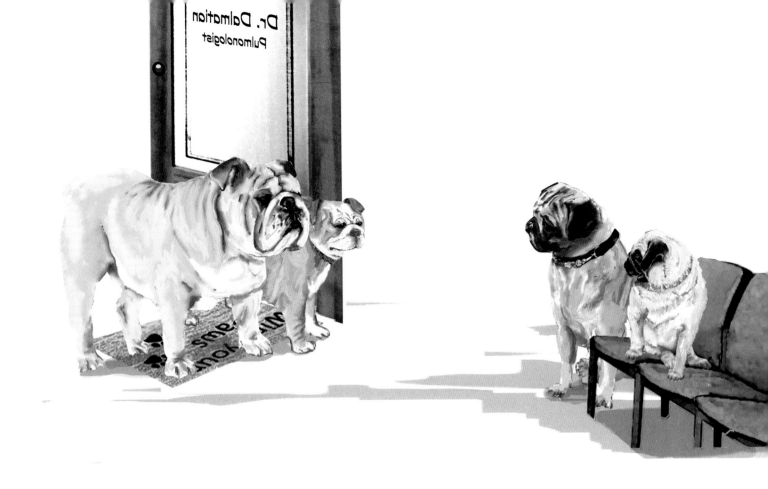

When Bina the Bulldog and her father walk into Dr. Dalmatian's office, she is surprised to see her classmate, Phoebe the Pug, sitting in the waiting room.

Bina is so frightened about what is happening to her, she doesn't make fun of Phoebe at all.

Phoebe the Pug notices how frightened Bina looks. Phoebe walks over and nicely says, "Why are you here, Bina?"

Bina the Bulldog says, "I am having trouble breathing. I went to the nurse's office, and Mr. Dachshund said I needed to see Dr. Dalmatian. Mr. Dachshund said that I might have to use a rescue inhaler, but I'm scared."

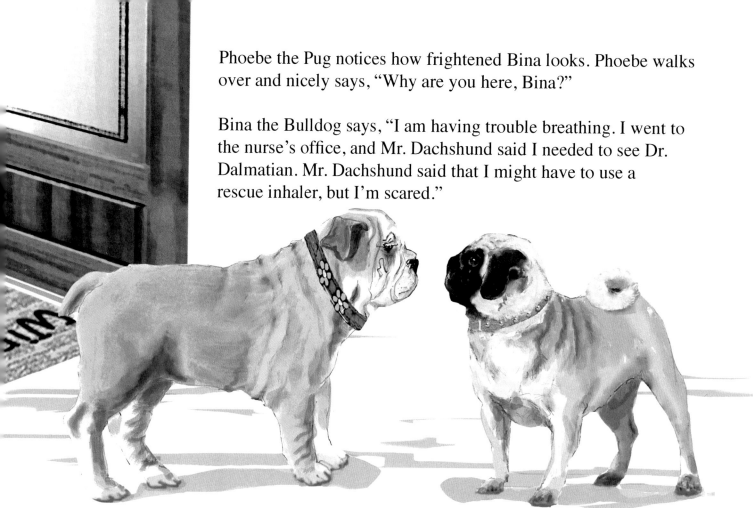

Phoebe gives an encouraging smile and says, "I use an emergency inhaler, and it isn't scary at all! It helps me breathe better. It might help you, too."

Bina says, "Why do you use it?"

Using a rescue inhaler isn't scary at all. And if you have asthma, you will need to carry one with you at all times. Going to see a specialist isn't scary either. Specialists know a lot about diseases and can help you feel better.

Phoebe the Pug says, "I use a rescue inhaler because I have asthma. Asthma sometimes makes it hard for my lungs and bronchial air passages to work properly. Bronchial air passages look like small branches in the lungs."

Phoebe encourages Bina, "Once you use your rescue inhaler, your breathing will be back to normal. And then you can play again. You don't have to be afraid of it."

She continues, "All of us have lungs and bronchial air passages, but not all of us have asthma."

Bina then asks, "What are you doing here?"

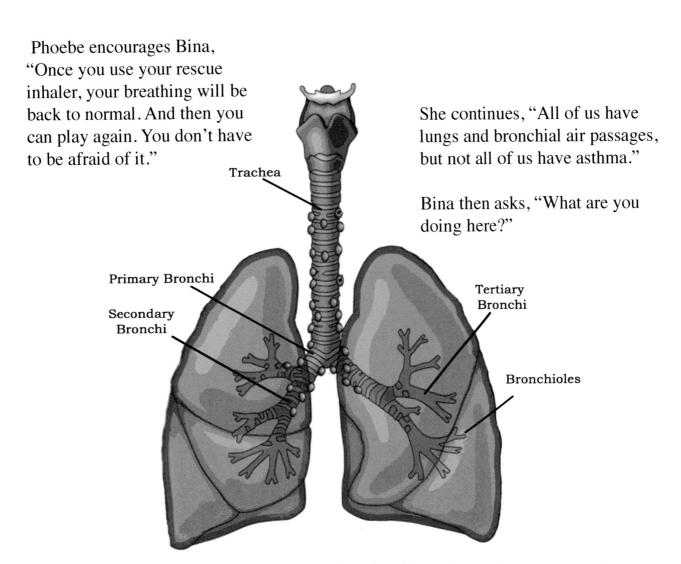

Trachea

Primary Bronchi

Secondary Bronchi

Tertiary Bronchi

Bronchioles

Phoebe replies, "I'm here to see Dr. Dalmatian. I continue to have more and more asthmatic episodes. I start to cough and wheeze, and sometimes I can't stop."

Bina chimes in and says, "Wheezing? That's what Mr. Dachshund said he heard in my lungs!"

Phoebe says, "Maybe you have asthma, too?"

Just then, Dr. Dalmatian comes out and says, "Phoebe, I'm ready for you."

Phoebe turns to Bina and says, "I hope you feel better soon." Bina smiles at her kindness and feels relieved. Phoebe's explanation helped her better understand what might be happening to her.

In the exam room, Phoebe tells Dr. Dalmatian about all the frequent asthmatic episodes she has had during the last few days and nights. He tells her that he will perform a series of tests to see what is triggering her asthma attacks.

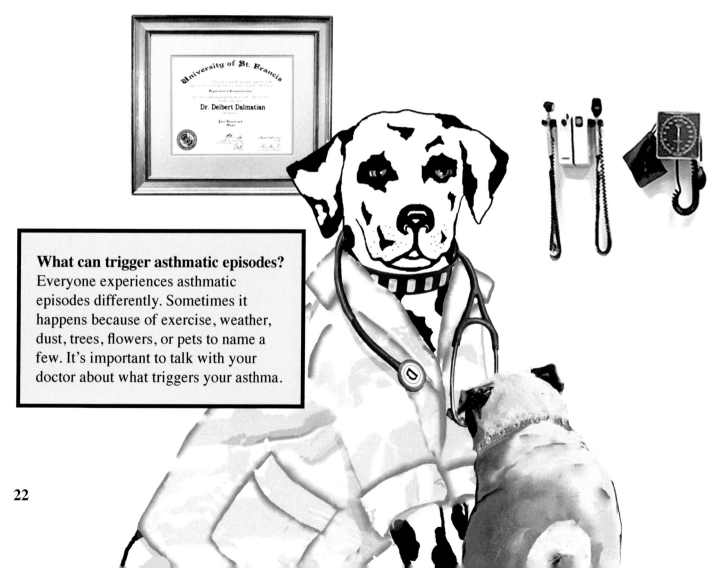

What can trigger asthmatic episodes?
Everyone experiences asthmatic episodes differently. Sometimes it happens because of exercise, weather, dust, trees, flowers, or pets to name a few. It's important to talk with your doctor about what triggers your asthma.

First, Dr. Dalmatian performs a Pulmonary Function Test. This test measures how well the lungs are working. Phoebe breathes into a mouthpiece that is connected to a large machine. It measures different things about her breathing.

Then Dr. Dalmatian presses a couple buttons on the machine. He says that he will be doing another test called, Spirometry. It measures how fast air flows in and out of her lungs. Phoebe continues to breathe into the mouthpiece connected to the machine.

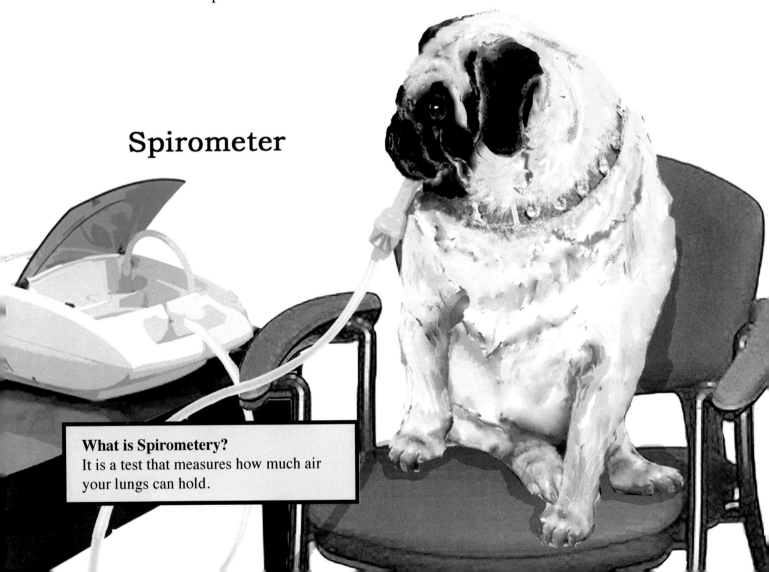

Spirometer

What is Spirometery?
It is a test that measures how much air your lungs can hold.

Dr. Dalmatian proceeds to perform a third test called an Exhaled Nitric Oxide Test. He gives Phoebe a different mouthpiece connected to a smaller machine. She blows into the mouthpiece steadily for several seconds. It measures how much of this chemical, called nitric oxide, is coming from her lungs. The more nitric oxide measured, the more irritated and inflamed her lungs are.

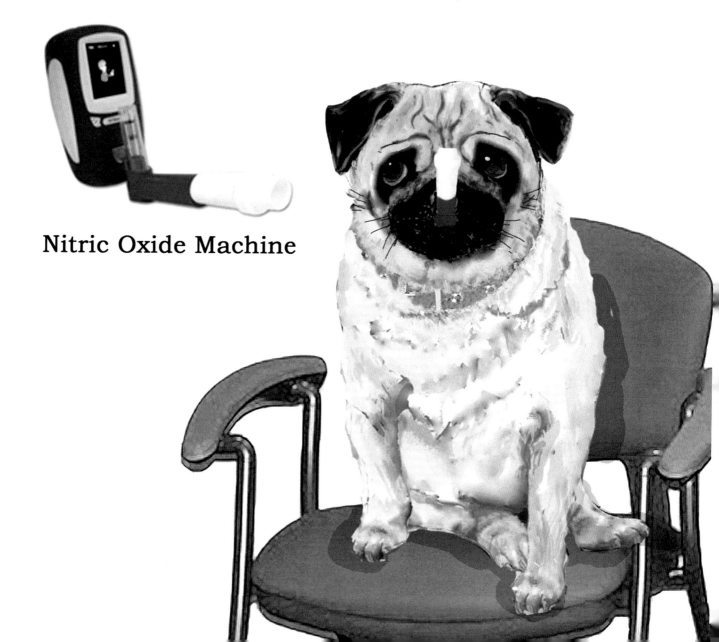

Nitric Oxide Machine

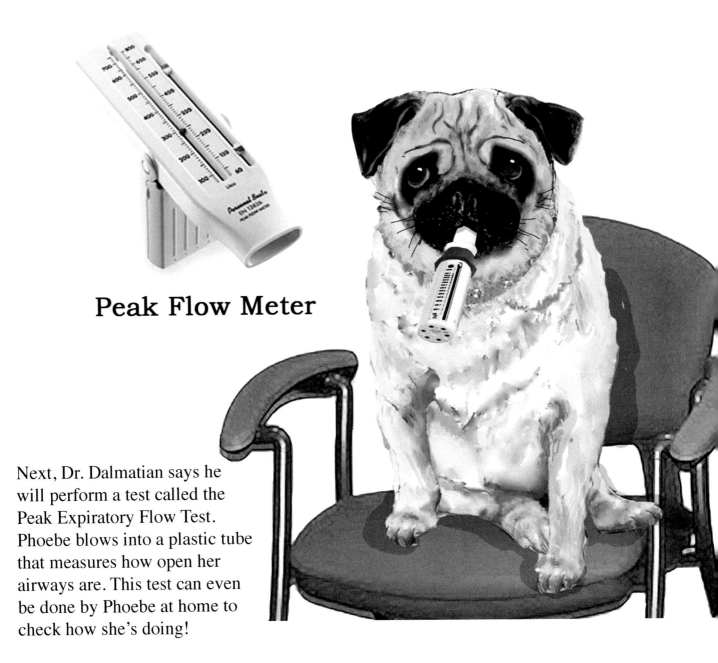

Peak Flow Meter

Next, Dr. Dalmatian says he will perform a test called the Peak Expiratory Flow Test. Phoebe blows into a plastic tube that measures how open her airways are. This test can even be done by Phoebe at home to check how she's doing!

Finally, he tests for allergies, or asthmatic triggers, by taking a blood sample and by performing a Skin Prick Test (also called a scratch test) on her skin to see what possible allergies may be causing her frequent asthmatic episodes.

25

After the tests are completed, she waits with her mom for the results.

A short while later, Dr. Dalmatian calls her back into the exam room and says, "Phoebe, based on your frequent symptoms and the test results, you have severe asthma. Don't worry, you are still a normal dog. It just means you need different medications to take care of yourself."

Dr. Dalmatian proceeds to explain how to control her severe asthma. He says that she will need to start using an additional inhaler on a regular basis. This additional inhaler is called a corticosteroid inhaler. It is used to help prevent asthmatic episodes from happening. She will still have a rescue inhaler and her nebulizer treatments to use as needed.

Phoebe is relieved that she now knows how to prevent many future asthmatic episodes.

Dr. Dalmatian says that as long as she follows his instructions, she will be able to be her old self again and play with the other pups at school.

What is a corticosteroid inhaler?
A corticosteroid inhaler is a medication that helps reduce inflammation in the lungs. There are three different ways people with asthma receive corticosteroids: through an inhaler, through a pill they swallow, or through a nose spray.

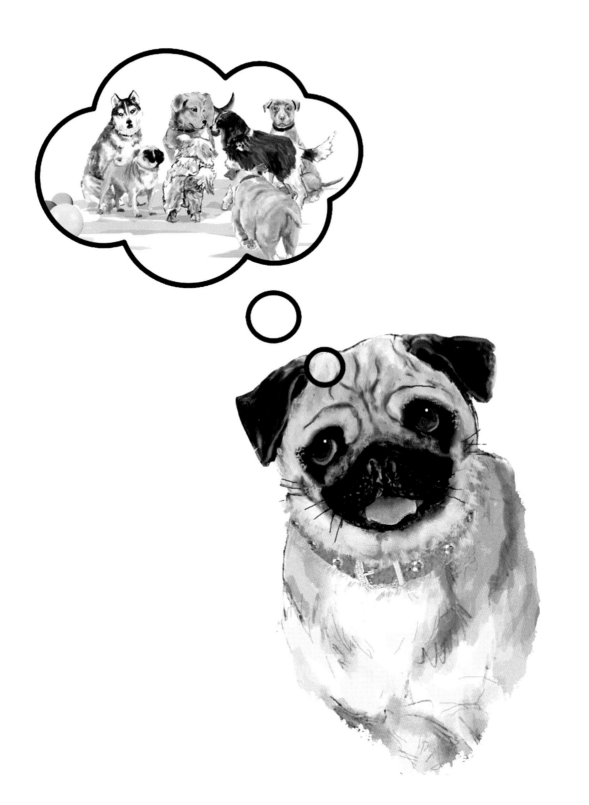

The next day, Phoebe goes back to school and sees Bina the Bulldog. At first, she is unsure if she should approach Bina. But then Bina runs up to Phoebe with her tail wagging and asks, "How did your exam go?"

Phoebe tells her that she has severe asthma, but she now has the medicine to help her feel better. Phoebe then asks, "How was your exam? Do you feel better today?"

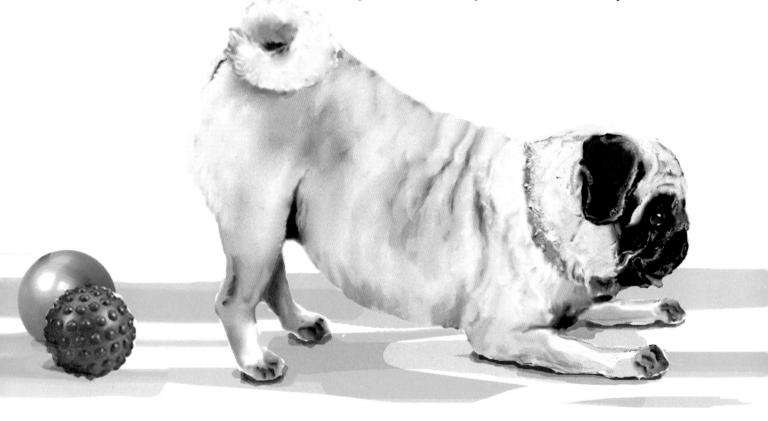

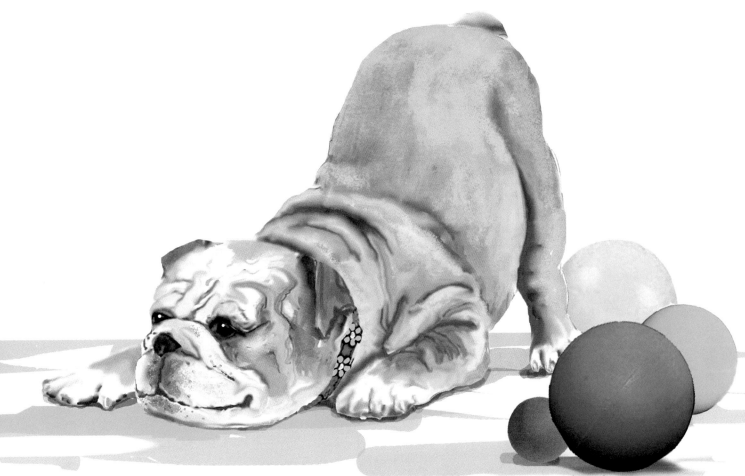

Bina answers, "Dr. Dalmatian said that I have mild asthma. For now, I just have to carry my rescue inhaler and use it when I need to. Thank you for sharing your experience with me and helping me feel brave. I did not understand what was happening to you. I now know the coughing and wheezing was not because you were sick. It's not your fault that you have asthma. I'm sorry I treated you badly. Hey! Do you want to come play with us today?"

Phoebe is so happy that she wags her tail and barks, "Sure!"

29

Parents/Teachers & Kids Discussion Area

Bina the Bulldog bullied Phoebe the Pug in the beginning of the story. How can you recognize and help prevent bullying?

What are some examples of how to stop bullying?

When Phoebe had an asthmatic episode in the playground, what did the other pups do? What can they do differently next time?

Phoebe was very sad and embarrassed because of her coughing and wheezing. How can you help her not feel sad and embarrassed?

What did Bina the Bulldog learn about the proper way to treat others who are different?

Asthma & Bullying

1 in 10 children with asthma report bullying or teasing related to their condition.

Signs that your child may be at risk for bullying:

- Your child displays an abrupt lack of interest in school or refuses to attend school.
- Your child suffers a drop in his/her grades.
- Your child withdraws from family and/or school activities
- He/she may want to be left alone.
- Your child is taking your money and making poor excuses for where it went.
- Your child is sad, sullen, angry or scared after using the phone or Internet.
- Your child stops talking about their peers and everyday activities.
- Your child has physical injuries not consistent with an explanation.
- Your child has stomachaches, headaches, and panic attacks.
- He/she may be unable to sleep, sleep too much or is exhausted.

For help or guidance:

www.bullying.org
www.lfcc.on.ca/bully.htm
www.opheliaproject.org
www.stopbullyingnow.com

Sometimes mild asthma may progressively become severe asthma.

You may need to see an asthma specialist, also known as a pulmonologist, if you have had one or more of the following experiences:

- Have poorly controlled asthma
- Have needed treatment with oral corticosteroids (such as prednisone) more than once in the past year
- Have had daytime symptoms and nighttime awakenings more than two times a month
- Have had trouble breathing during physical activities
- Have been missing multiple days of school (or work) due to asthmatic symptoms or episodes
- Have had to visit the emergency room or hospital more than once in the past year for breathing problems
- Have needed to be in the intensive care unit for breathing issues
- Are not responding to or are having side effects from medications

For help or guidance:

http://severeasthmafoundation.com/
http://www.allergyasthmanetwork.org/
http://www.upmc.com/Services/pulmonology/asthma/Pages/default.aspx
http://www.thoracic.org/
https://www.cdc.gov/asthma/default.htm
http://www.chestnet.org/Foundation
https://www.aaaai.org/

Persistent signs and symptoms like coughing and wheezing may signal a possible greater issue. Seek medical attention to address symptoms before they get worse.

A cough is not always "just a cough".

All asthma is not the same. Diagnosis involves careful consideration of the patient's medical history, physical exam, and laboratory tests.

Made in the USA
Lexington, KY
19 December 2019

58684753R00024